Hugh Nepis

Is That a Gun in Your Pocket?

A compendium for the well-endowed man

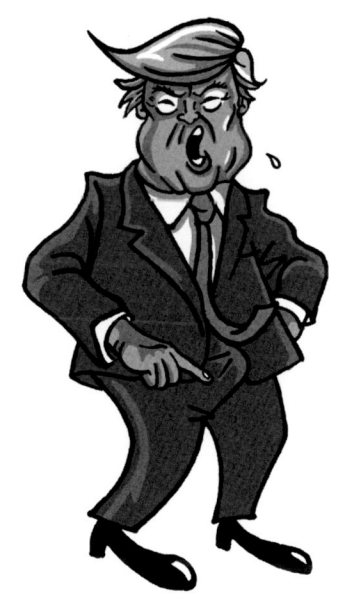

novum pro

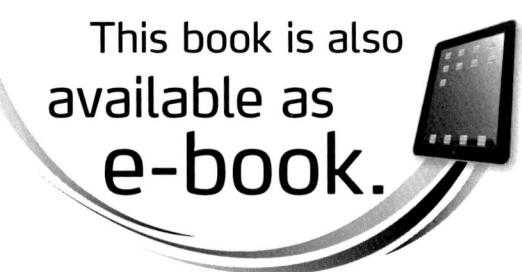

www.novum-publishing.co.uk

All rights of distribution, including via film, radio, and television, photomechanical reproduction, audio storage media, electronic data storage media, and the reprinting of portions of text, are reserved.

Printed in the European Union on environmentally friendly, chlorine- and acid-free paper.

© 2021 novum publishing

ISBN 978-3-99107-161-7
Editing: Hugo Chandler, BA
Cover photo: Bernie Lee
Cover design, layout & typesetting: novum publishing
Internal illustrations:
Bernie Lee & Hugh Nepis

www.novum-publishing.co.uk

ACKNOWLEDGEMENT

I would like to thank Dan and Jean for sullying their artistic integrity by being the first to read an edit of the original copy of this sordid little book.

This book is for adults, though parents may want to use it as a colouring book for their children.

HOW TO HANDLE A LARGE PENIS

A fellow took my photograph it cost one and three.
I said when it was done, "Is that supposed to be me?"
"You've properly mucked it up the only thing I can see is
My little stick of Blackpool Rock."

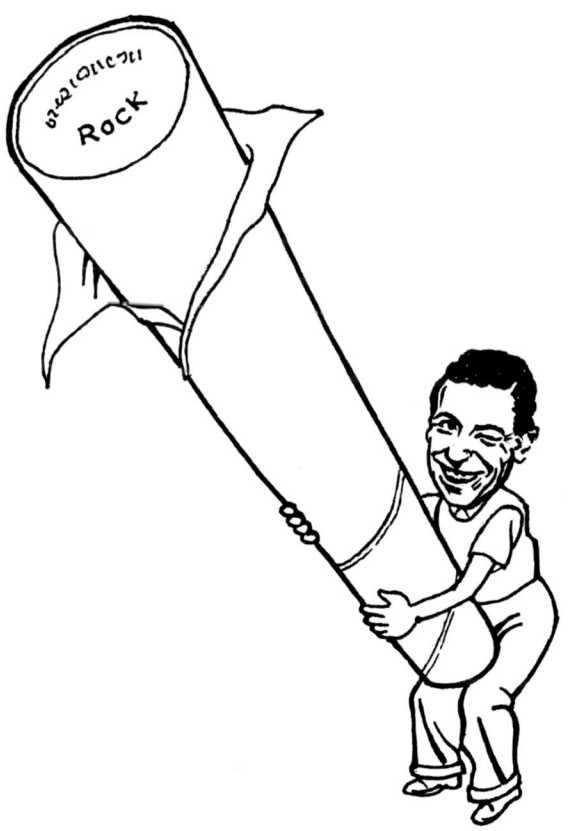

When I told my friends that I was going to write a book on men with large penises, they weren't shocked but amused and maybe bemused. They all agreed that if anyone were capable of writing such a book it would be me. My problem was how to approach it, I knew I wanted it to be partly satirical, partly informative and just slightly serious. I also wanted cartoons to highlight the satire, and that it should be approached from both a gay and a heterosexual perspective. My first consideration was defining a large penis.

Are men really that interested in the size of their penis? Well, according to World Data no other topic on their website has been asked for more often, than the average size of the penis. So, I guess the answer is yes. But why? – is it because it helps to improve their status? makes them more manly? helps them to feel secure? Or is it a feeling of inadequacy? After reading this book I doubt if you'll still be able to answer the question of why, but it's a fun read.

What is our point of reference?

To talk about a large penis, one has to establish first of all what we are referring to as large. Is it cucumber size or toilet roll size? For the purposes of this book we will base it on accepted data. Four to six inches is considered the average size of a man's penis in the UK. Over six inches is thought to be large; between eight and ten is extra-large. Over ten inches is very rare, and not part of this book's remit. Circumference is also important: a large penis is somewhere in the region of five to six inches all the way round, though of course there can be variations on that.

How is the penis measured? According to the World Data website, the length is always measured from the top of the stem root to the top of the glans. The measurement of the circumference is usually taken at the root.

MAN'S OWN PERCEPTION OF HIS GENITALIA

I read a book recently on how men with large penises can be self-conscious and neurotic. I have to say that I have never come across this condition; on the contrary, men with over-developed genitalia seem, on the whole, to be rather proud of it and tend to boast about it.

MICRO/MACROPENISES

Micropenises are abnormally small, and to understand the problems and advantages of a large penis we should briefly examine those with undersized cocks. I think where the problem in penis size is more apparent is with men with small, almost pre-puberty penises. The novelist and short story writer Franz Kafka is known to have had neurosis about the size of his dick, as did Scott Fitzgerald. I have known guys in the past with small appendages who have tried to draw attention to them by having them tattooed or having a piercing across the urethra called a Prince Albert; very painful, I imagine, and it would have the effect of making you piss like a watering can.

A gay friend of mine with a very small penis and who was also into S&M was told by his master or controller that he should be ashamed of possessing such a small cock and had him lock it away in a chastity cage, with the key being held by his controller. This must have done wonders for his self-esteem.

Such behaviour as this I have never known to be reported by men with large dicks. This condition is known as a macropenis or megaopenis. Some babies are delivered with a large phallus, or it enlarges rapidly in childhood, resulting from high levels of testosterone.

Some men opt for penis reduction purely for sexual pleasure; either for themselves or for their sexual partner.

THE PENIS IN HISTORY

The large penis has always been a factor in male masculinity. As far back as the Greeks, Priapus, the god of male genitalia, was always depicted by his large and oversized permanent erection. Apollo, the most beautiful of the gods, was supposed to have a large dick, making all the other gods envious and resentful.

Greek drama certainly featured the large penis. One only has to consider the comedies of Aristophanes. The men would strap on very large penises and cavort around the stage in a very lewd and crude manner. There was nothing subtle about the Greeks. Their appetite and lust for all that was crude was satisfied only by the actors' actions. For them, the coarser the better.

The Romans adopted many Greek Gods. One in particular was Priapus, the god not only of farm animals but also male genitalia. In the House of Casa dei Vetti in Pompi he is depicted with an over-sized penis, which is permanently erect. (It can't have done much for his heart.). Priapus is seen in much of Roman art, though one image stands out where his penis is being weighed for a bag of gold, giving rise to the expression 'worth its weight in gold'.

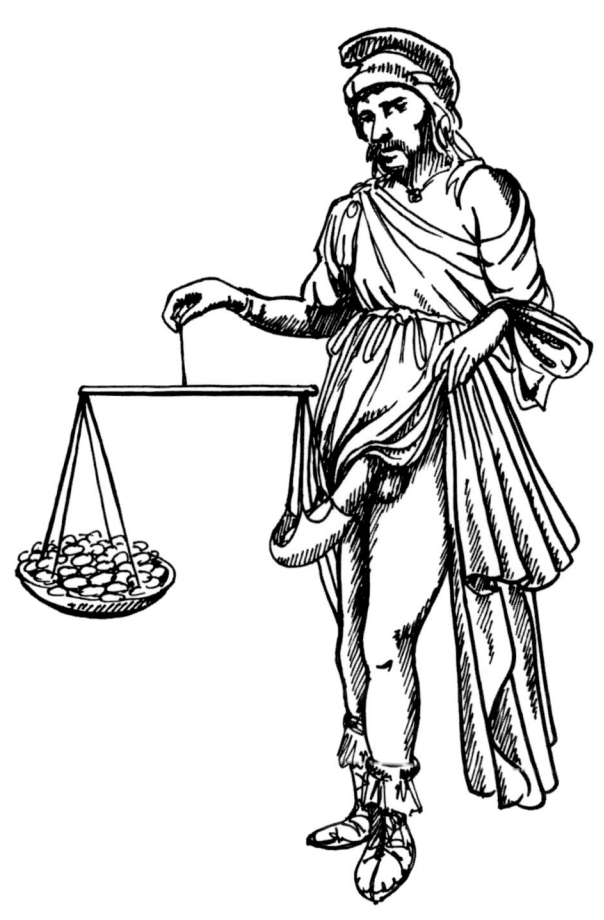

'Worth its weight in gold'

In Roman times, you only have to look at the Walls of Pompeii to realise how they revered the male genitalia. Mind you, the Romans were a perverted lot. During the reigns of Nero and Commodus, the use of the penis as a means of amusement to satisfy the Roman crowds in the arena was quite common. There was nothing more fun than to have a woman tied to a post in the middle of the arena to see how large a penis she could take.

For real fun, they would have her raped by baboons, monkeys, and then, for a laugh, a donkey. As the girl screamed before she passed out, the audience would cheer. It would, of course, have traumatised the girl, but mercifully, at the end of the ordeal, they would cut her throat. So, the Romans did have a heart after all.

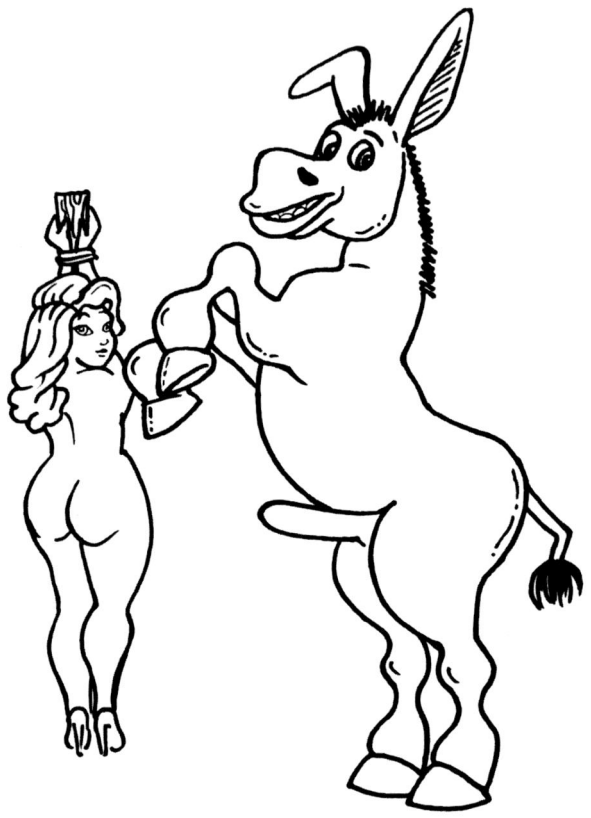

'I'm sure Muffin the Mule was never asked to do this'

Spartacus, who led the slave uprising, was supposedly well-endowed, as was Alexander the Great, and it wasn't just Rome that attracted Cleopatra to Anthony, but this of course is simply legend. The ancients liked to endow their heroes with such fanciful attributes as twenty-first century culture does with today's pop and film stars; but most of it is idle gossip and very little more than speculation.

During the Middle Ages men would wear a codpiece to cover their 'man of war'. Of course the sight of a larger and more bejewelled codpiece would inform a woman what sort of man she was dealing with, and he would find himself in the stocks for misrepresentation of merchandise if he didn't live up to the product he supposedly had on show.

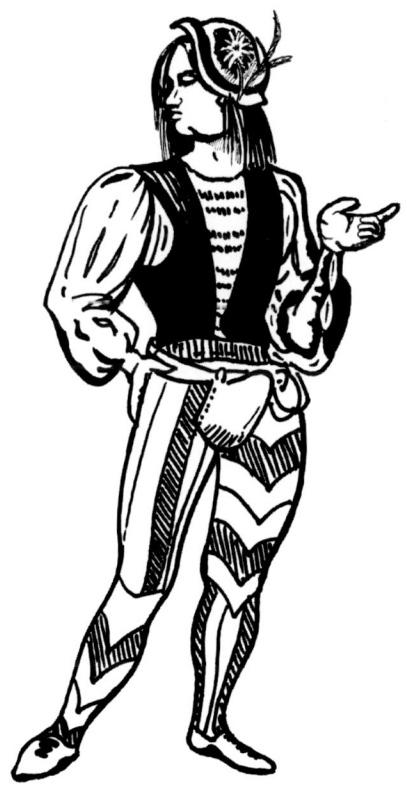

'I've got a noble cock it crows at break of day.' (Chaucer).

The eighteenth century was, I believe, the crudest period in European history. The exposure and flaunting of the penis were not uncommon. The fact that half of them were pox-ridden seemed to be of little concern to the ladies, whom these peacocks were trying to impress. They may have had powdered wigs and satin clothes, but their personal hygiene left much to be desired.

The reign of Victoria put a stop to all that crude vulgarity or did it? – not on your life; it simply drove it underground. The size of a man's penis became the butt of many a music-hall joke. Smutty or suggestive songs have always been a popular source of amusement, such as Stanley Smith Master's *The Marrow Song*.

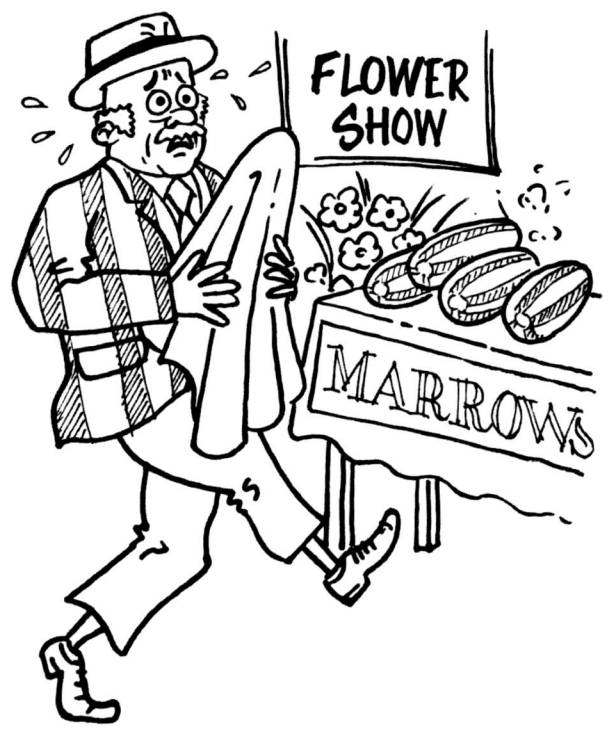

'Oh, what a beauty'

Oh, what a beauty,
I've never seen one as big as that before.
Oh, what a beauty,
It must be 6 foot long or even more.
It's such a lovely colour,
So big and round and fat.
I never knew a marrow could grow as big as that.

Then of course, there was George Formby's *With My Little Stick of Blackpool Rock*. Although the song never rhymes "rock" with the obvious, it really doesn't need an academic with a literature degree to explain the metaphorical significance of the small and sticky object in his pocket.

PUBERTY AND THE DEVELOPMENT OF THE MONSTER

Between the ages of twelve and fourteen, boys usually go through a period of puberty and penis development. It often happens without them really noticing it. I have to say I wasn't aware of my own growth. Maybe it would have been different if I'd been at a British public school where Elliot Minor's cock was on public display,

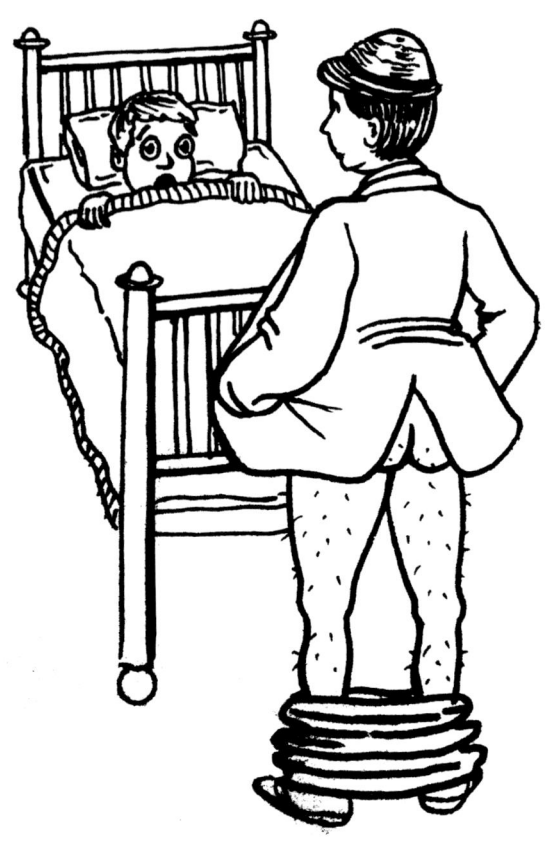

'I say, Elliot minor that's a stinker'

I might have realised the growth in myself. Sadly, such privilege was not awarded to me. It wasn't until I was fourteen and played the game *I'll show you mine if you show me yours* with another boy that I realised what I had in my pants. He got his out first and then I produced mine. "Fuck," he exclaimed, "that's huge."

I didn't believe it was, but it was only then that I realised that boys developed cock sizes at different rates. Now, according to the book I read at Christmas, I should have been embarrassed and self-conscious. I wasn't in the least. In fact, I was rather proud.

Large penises and erections can be very difficult to handle during adolescence. I remember at the age of fifteen travelling on a tube to Piccadilly. With the vibration of the train, unfortunate things started happening in my pants. When we got to Piccadilly, I couldn't stand up to get off the Tube. I had to travel all the way to Holborn before it subsided. I got off the train self-consciously and then I had to travel back to my appointment in Piccadilly.

PROBLEMS WITH A LARGE PENIS

There is, however, a serious side to the size of the penis. It can cause serious concerns to some men if it's considered too big. Will my partner be able to take it? Should I see a doctor? I'm not sure you can have a penis reduction. The fact is that a very large penis can do very little harm. Even when it's hard and erect it is only made up of soft tissue and will give way to any orifice it may be inserted into. It can, however, be off-putting and daunting, and for the participant, be it male or female, it can be frightening and painful. The recommended way to first initiate intercourse is for the man to lay on the bed with his penis erect and for the partner to slowly lower on to it. By doing this, the participant is taking control and allowing the insertion to happen on their terms. After a period of sexual intercourse in this way, normal activities can be resumed.

It always amuses me when women try to get a divorce on the grounds that their husband's penis is too large. Didn't she check it out before the wedding night? A simple grope would have told her. The wife's argument falls at the first fence, however, when she produces her children. Were they produced by some form of immaculate conception? Or is it being suggested that Joseph was also well-hung?

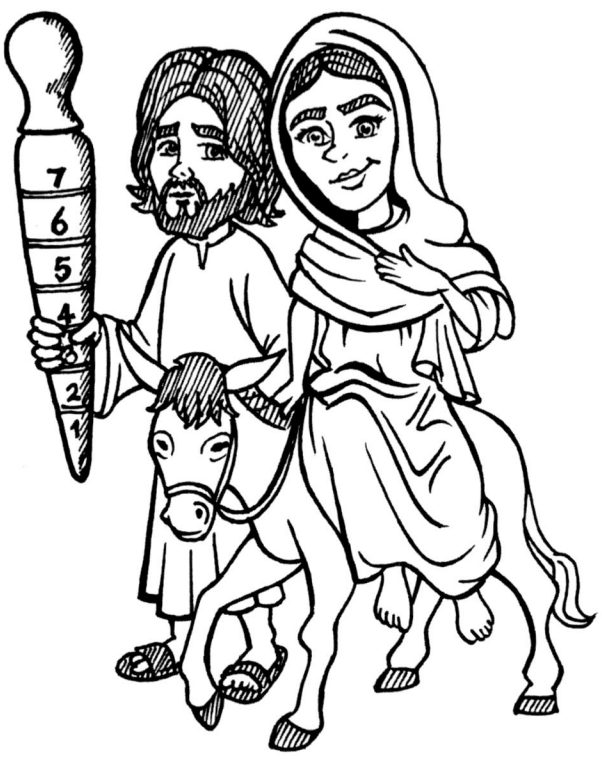

'I know you're a carpenter but do you have to use such a big tool'.

WHAT TO WEAR

Of course, there is the popular adage: 'If you've got it, flaunt it'. The chav in his jogging bottoms with no underwear, letting the world see he's a swinging guy. If you want to attract the ladies with your extra accoutrements, then make sure you pay and display. In the swimming pool never hide your bushel in boxer swimming gear; wear tight black trunks, I mean just look what it did for Tom Daley.

BIG COCKS AND CELEBS

Many celebrities of course brag about their large appendages. Top of the list is Donald Trump, or is it just fake news? He tells us that the ladies like his large modus operandi. I think they are more likely to appreciate his large bank account.

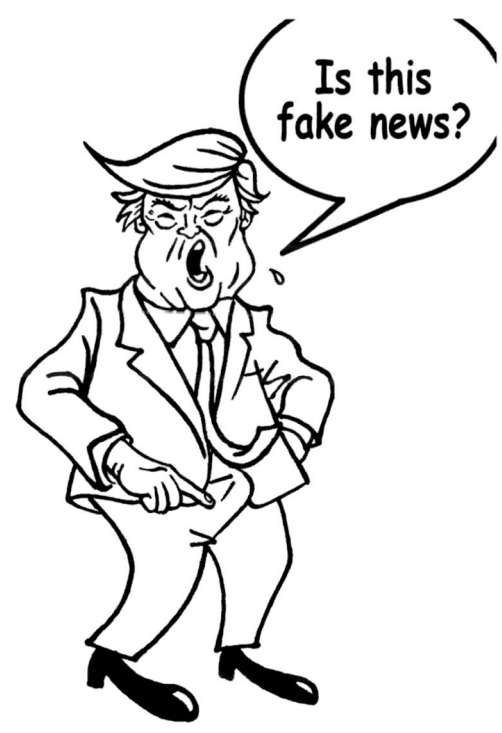

'Is this fake news?'

Another celebrity, not known for his looks, was Andrew Lloyd Webber, who was outed as being one of the big boys by his ex-wife Sarah Brightman. Andrew then confirmed this on the Jonathan Ross show. Good for you, Andrew.

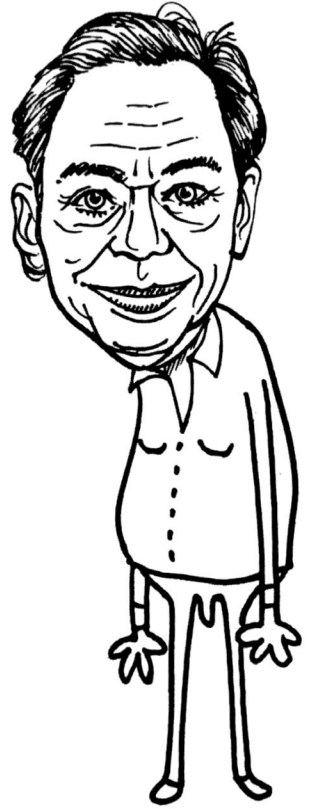

'Love changes everything'

Even 'Strictly Come Dancing' had its moments of penis revelations when all the male dancers in their mature and sensible way chose to have a competition on who had the biggest cock. It is understood that AJ Pritchard won the competition but as no one can verify it, we'll have to leave it pending.

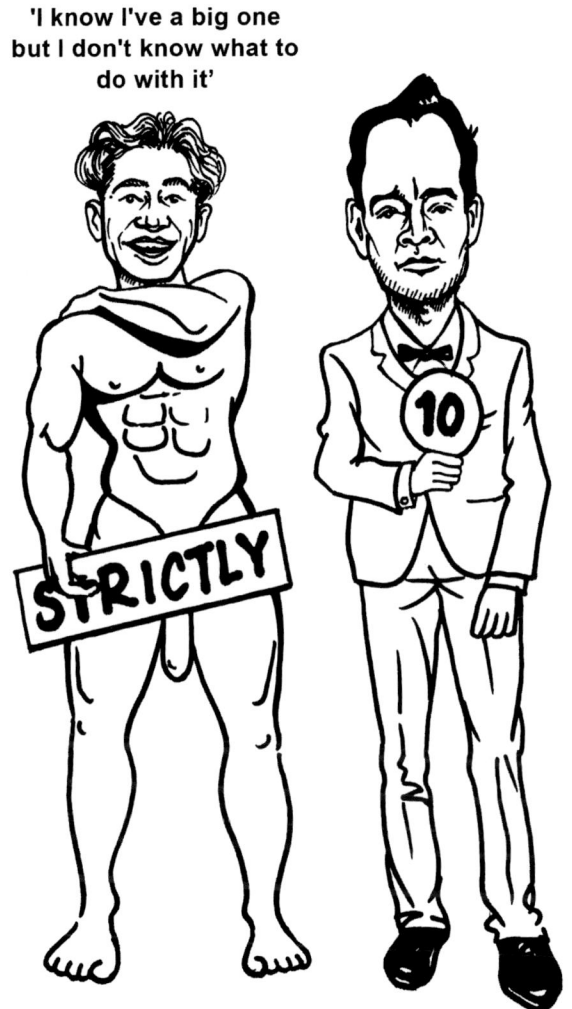

Hollywood celebs and superstars are often reported as being well endowed. Here's the top twenty:

1. Rudolph Nureyev, the international ballet dancer, was known for his nine-inch penis. The bulge in his tights would suggest that it is true.
2. Errol Flynn (1940s film star); known for his flashy cutlass when on the Spanish Main.
3. Matt Baker (presenter of 'The One Show' and 'Country File'). One only had to see him in the Palladium Pantomime in his mankini to see that Matt is no shy guy.
4. Andrew Lloyd Webber, whose musical instrument is supposedly able to stretch a whole octave (I think there may be a slight exaggeration there).
5. Jason Momoa ('Game of Thrones'). He looks like a mean brute of a man, but the brute lies below.
6. Tom Daley likes to be photographed showing his prowess.
7. David Beckham (footballer and model for Emporio Armani). He modelled in tight white underwear for Armani as he needed the money.
8. Mick Jagger; supposedly a good seven inches. The way he's gyrated his hips during his life is bound to have kept it stimulated.
9. James Norton (star of 'War and Peace' and the TV series 'Granchester'). He's not just good-looking and a good actor. He evidently has other features that make him stand out.
10. Daniel Craig. Judy Dench described it as an absolute monster. Good for you Judy! 'There is nothing like a Dame'.
11. A.J Pritchard won the biggest size in Strictly.
12. Rick Edwards (host of 'Impossible!'). Is his 10 inches really 'Impossible!'
13. Chris Hughes (of 'Love Island' fame). It was suggested that he had over nine inches of raw fresh meat between his legs (made him sound like a butcher).
14. Prince Charles. I wonder if he inherited more than his title from his great-great-great-grandfather, Prince Albert.

15. Brandon Myers ('Bromans' reality show). With his dick that reaches the bottom of a pint beer glass, Brandon thinks he can challenge Chris Hughes.
16. Justin Bieber (pop star) – exposed himself on holiday with Jayde Pierce at Bora Bora. Surprise! Surprised the paparazzi were around? – his exhibitionism knows no bounds.
17. David Hasselhoff (star of 'Bay Watch'). With his man of war, even the sharks dive for cover.
18. Cristiano Ronaldo. He posed naked with his girlfriend, Irina, on the front cover of Vogue España. Though one doesn't see his essentials, you wouldn't go naked unless you had something to be proud of.
19. Orlando Bloom was angry when photographed by the world press while skinny-dipping in Sardinia – well, what did he expect?
20. Eddie Murphy. Gary Griffin, author of *Penis Size and Enlargement* describes Murphy as being 'very well-equipped' – probably in the eight to nine inch range; very much the donkey.

All these comments are nothing more than London and Hollywood gossip. The question that must be asked of the people who reported the sizes is: How the hell did they know? I can believe that some were indiscreet when swimming on holiday. I can even see it through ill-considered photographs. But I find it hard to believe that an actor would walk on to a film set with his manhood exposed for all the film crew to see.

ROYAL COCKS AND CANAPES

From William I to the present day, English kings have not been known for their appendages. They have no problem producing the next royal issue but on size they're way down the pecking order, with the exception of Prince Albert who astounded Queen

Victoria with his German donger. Mind you – poor cow – she'd never seen an erect penis until her wedding night.

But if we look over the water to Europe, we will discover one country that did have a monarch with something of a size problem. King Ferdinand VII of Spain (1784–1833) was not only exceedingly plain – as seen in the portrait by Goya – and not only was he a bad and corrupt ruler, but he was also the possessor of a ginormous penis. And the king's dick wasn't just very large. It was also deformed, starting with a thin root and expanding into a large bulbous cock. Due to the size and deformity of the product he was unable to produce children to his first three wives.

For his fourth wife, Maria Christina, he thought 'enough is enough' and had a special cushion made to help him impregnate the queen. The cushion supported the narrow base, leaving only the bulbous tip to bob above the parapet. Thus allowing the queen to straddle it. This she did and produced a daughter who later became Isabel II of Spain. When the king paraded down the corridors of power his subjects bowing low would be heard to mumble: 'God save the king! … and god help the queen.'

Now I bet you didn't learn these facts in your history lesson.

Mae West once said in a film 'Is that a gun in your pocket or are you just pleased to see me?' It's a funny line with an underlying truth. There is an expression 'an erect penis has no conscience', and it's true. How many men have got themselves into trouble by being ruled by their dick? This, of course, doesn't just apply to men with big cocks. Indeed, the larger the cock, the harder it is to sustain a strong erection. The blood pumping round a nine-incher can affect a man's blood pressure, and therefore his desire is often curtailed before he can get himself into any real trouble.

MYTHS AND BRAGGING

There have developed over the years several myths indicating the size of a man's penis. The size of his feet ... has he a big nose? ... look at his hands ... etc. It's clearly shown that none of these indicators is in any way correct. There is, however, a correlation regarding the size of your penis and where you actually come from. So, there is some truth in saying black men have big cocks. A survey done for the *Journal of Urology* showed that the largest penises were attributed to men in Africa and South America, whereas those born in Asia had smaller genitalia than men born in Europe. Sadly, those in the UK and the USA come way down the chart.

It must be pointed out that this survey is at its heart flawed, as in some cases there were only a few dozen test persons in a country, which doesn't allow for a representative survey. Measurements were, however, only allowed where they had, in the words of 'Strictly Come Dancing', been externally verified. That must have been a fun job for someone. So, the chart below, though interesting, only gives an indication of size related to areas of the world and should not be considered as absolute.

PENIS SIZES BY COUNTRY OF ORIGIN

Country	Erect length in centimetres
1. Democratic Republic of the Congo	17.93
2. Ecuador	17.61
3. Cameroon	16.67
4. Bolivia	16.51
5. Sudan	16.47
6. Haiti	16.01

7.	Senegal	15.89
8.	Gambia	15.88
9.	Cuba	15.87
10.	Netherlands	15.87
11.	Zambia	15.78
12.	France	15.74
13.	Angola	15.73
14.	Italy	15.73
15.	Canada	15.71
16.	Egypt	15.69
17.	Zimbabwe	15.68
18.	Georgia	15.61
19.	Paraguay	15.53
20.	Chad	15.33
21.	Central African Republic	15.33
22.	Sweden	15.08
23.	Brazil	15.22
24.	Ivory Coast	15.22
25.	Bulgaria	15.02
26.	Costa Rica	15.01
27.	Honduras	15.00
28.	Hungary	14,99
29.	Mexico	14.92
30.	Denmark	14.88
31.	Argentina	14.88
32.	El Salvador	14.88
33.	Serbia	14.87
34.	Belgium	14.77
35.	Latvia	14.69
36.	Belarus	14.63
37.	Chile	14.59
38.	Austria	14.53
39.	Germany	14.52
40.	Algeria	14.49
41.	Australia	14.46

42. Nigeria   14.38
43. Switzerland   14.35
44. Norway   14,34
45. Poland   14.29
46. Albania   14.19
47. New Zealand   13.99
48. North Macedonia   13.98
49. Ukraine   13.97
50. Spain   13.85
51. Finland   13.77
52. Libya   13.74
53. Azerbaijan   13,72
54. Afghanistan   13.69
55. Israel   13.60
56. United States   13.58
57. Japan   13.56
58. Turkmenistan   13.48
59. Russia   13.21
60. South Korea   13.16
61. Armenia   13.14
62. United Kingdom   13.13
63. Ireland   12.78
64. Mongolia   12.77
65. Romania   12.73
66. Yemen   12.72
67. Pakistan   12,20
68. China   12.11
69. Indonesia   11,67
70. Singapore   11.53
71. Malaysia   11.49
72. Vietnam   11.47
73. Thailand   11.45
74. Bangladesh   11.20
75. Hong Kong   11.19
76. Sri Lanka   10.89
77. Philippines   10.85

78. Taiwan   10.78
79. Burma   10.70
80. Cambodia   10.04

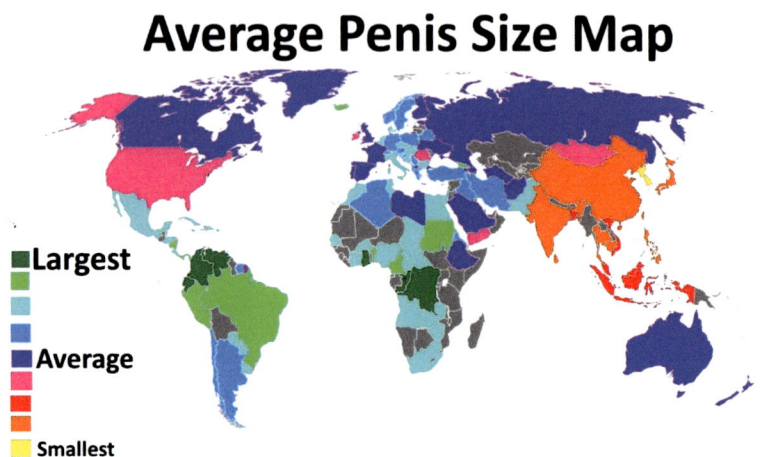

MALE PORN STARS AND THEIR STUDIOS

During the 1980s/90s, Jonah Adam (Cardeli) Falcon gave his name to a porn distribution site producing videos and magazines of an explicit nature, for the gay as well as the heterosexual market. Falcon, as he likes to be known, came to prominence when it was reported that the size of his penis was the largest in the world, measuring 13.5 inches. This record was challenged by South American Roberto Esquivel Cabrera swinging into the ring with a donger of 18.9 inches. Falcon maintained that Roberto cheated by stretching his genitalia using weights. (Ouch!).

A court case ensued, proving the importance of size in the porn industry.

I feel we cannot leave the subject of porn without mentioning Jeff Stryker. Here was a really good-looking porn star with a beautifully formed 9-inch penis. He didn't need to muddy the water on size; he had his own fan club. Both the ladies and the men loved his looks and adored his armoury. He had a dildo modelled on his penis, the 'Jeff Striker cock', which had major sales in the sex toy world.

BUKKAKEBOYS.COM

I went to a small gathering the other night and it was suggested we play a game called 'Cards Against Humanity'. Definitely not a PC game. It's a card game where every person is given ten cards with outrageous words written on. One of the group takes a card with a statement written on it, and everyone then has to offer one of their cards as the most outrageous response.

On this particular evening, Jenny picked a statement card and looked at it with great puzzlement. She then announced with complete innocence, 'What does Bukkake mean?'

The room fell silent, a few restrained giggles and then Simon answered by telling her to look it up on the internet when she got home. If she eventually did, she would have found the answer to be 'a sexual act where a group of men ejaculate over someone's face.' You may find this shocking and disgusting, which I understand, but you have a choice: Don't go on to the site or switch it off.

The word 'bukkake' comes to us from the Japanese for 'to sprinkle with water'. The Americans have certainly put their own spin on this definition. The centre of the Bukkake industry is in Los Angeles (where else?) and the company producing the videos is bukkakeboys.com. I mention the name because they're certainly not shy of their product. During the twenty-minute film they mention their name half a dozen times. I did find that the producers have a very unusual approach to pornographic films. For the first five minutes set in a lovely summer Hollywood garden, they interview the model who is to be the subject of the act. They ask completely innocuous questions: where he or she is from, what hobbies they have, do they like sport etc. They then if the models know what to expect when they enter 'the house'. Obviously, they do and it is only then that one of the guys who will be participating in the event conducts them inside.

In the room there are about twelve men with large erections ready for the Bukkake act. I have to say there is no roughness – no aggression or pinning the person down. Indeed, they project a party atmosphere and you do feel that the victim could get up at any time and walk out. I'm not sure on watching it what I exactly thought of the soulless performance and who it was really meant to appeal to. The only thing I could think of was the word of the English comedienne Anna Russell when she described a form of singing to be rather like 'jugglers and conjurers – enough being definitely enough'.

You may wonder why I include this sensorial piece of literary description in my book on men's obsession with a large penis. I think it's partly because all the men had large penises and the very fact that they were performing the act in such a passionless way. I suspect that most of the men were straight, which is odd in itself. Twelve straight men making an obviously gay pornographic film. All I can say is that the pay must have been good.

It seemed to me that the whole bukkake performance was a celebration of the penis. There was no other sex taking place and the sole focus was the above-average members on display.

After watching the film where masturbation is taken down to the level of washing your hair or cleaning your teeth, I was drawn to ask one question: If all animals have sex, why is it that no other animal lays down and allows other animals to masturbate over them? Maybe because of our intelligence we demand heightened stimulation, but I couldn't really see any stimulation here. I'm sure Freud would have had an answer.

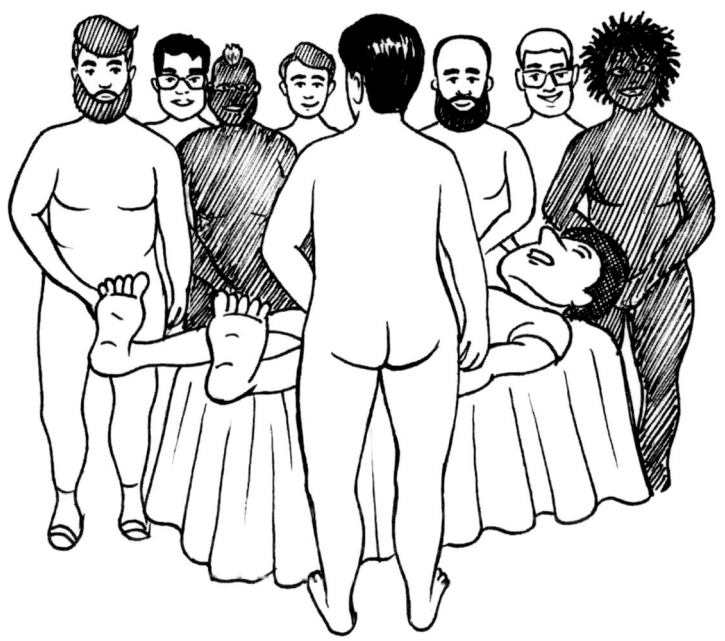

'Do you want raspberry or vanilla flavour?'

ANTISEMITISM AND THE POLITICISATION OF THE PENIS

I think it is time now, to be a little more serious. I was born in 1942, in the middle of the Second World War and went to the local infant school, which was in the middle of a somewhat deprived housing estate. Therefore, the comments I now make come directly from that working-class culture and the environment I was subjected to.

It's not in the remit of this book to be in any way political. There is, however, one area of penis culture that cannot be ignored. During the 1940s, the world was shocked by the atrocities perpetrated on the Jewish race during what was called the Holocaust. We condemn Nazi Germany for allowing this to happen, but this to an extent is unfair. Pre-1939, all of Europe suffered from anti-Semitic prejudice. It was not just Germany, but Poland, Russia, Czechoslovakia, and, sadly, Great Britain – particularly, it seemed, in the North East ports, where Jews escaping the Nazis passed through. After the war, though people were shocked and horrified at the Holocaust, the dark shadow of anti-Semitism still lurked in the back of the psyche – what if a Nazi regime should rise again? Based on these prejudices, many people refused to have their sons circumcised. Circumcision was the sure mark of a Jew. Parents didn't want their child to be seen in a PE lesson with a circumcised cock, fearing rumours of Jewish blood in the family. The fact that the foreskin could not be pulled back led to pain and discomfort for the child. Even recently, a parent told me that her nine-year-old son had to go into hospital for a circumcision and asked me not to tell anyone. It was said with almost a sense of shame.

During the 1950s and 1960s the gay community started to build up its own language called Polari. This is attributed mainly to a popular radio programme of the day called 'Round the Horn'. Gay patois, however, had its roots in the gay vernacular far earlier than when Kenneth Williams first espoused it. It was an attempt to make what may appear unsavoury activities more acceptable. For instance, a public convenience was a 'cottage', and if you came across a particularly attractive man you might comment, *'Vader their dolly old eek'. (Look at their pretty face.)*. My favourite cottaging polari however, was a 1950s northern expression for the pulling back of the foreskin on the penis, which was given the theatrical terms 'Drury Lane drapes' and 'Colosseum curtains'. If the curtains did not draw back, it was said that the curtain was down or closed. A more direct term for it was 'a blind cock', not a particularly nice expression but unambiguous in its meaning. You may ask why I include this in a book on the large penis. It is because when a boy reaches puberty the foreskin is stretched and can be very painful. It causes discomfort for the young man with a small or average penis, but so much more pain for a fellow with a big wanger.

In the multi-cultural Britain of today, circumcision is far more accepted, even though in recent times anti-Semitism and Islamophobia have raised their unpleasant heads. The truth is that the matter is one of cleanliness. North Africa is a dry, dust-and-sand ridden area of the world, and to have your son circumcised avoids irritation and infection. The Jews and the Muslims may like to regard it as part of their religious beliefs, but it really is nothing more than to show what clean people they are, much to the annoyance of European culture.

THE FSLP

During the 1960s, my friend and I joined, for a joke, an organisation called the FSLP which stood for the 'Foundation for the Support of the Large Penis'. I had to fill in a form and send it to somewhere in Aylesbury. The form asked for my name, address, age, and the size of my penis. I could have put any size; they wouldn't know. A month after sending my form and a postal order for five pounds, I received a tin badge, a certificate, and a list of rules, such as keep it clean, be proud of it, be discreet, etc. It really was quite absurd. Included in the package was a cheap handkerchief and an equally cheap sachet of hand lotion. Why, I have no idea. I realised then that it was a scam and a friend and

I, much to my regret now, threw the articles away. I suspect I'd get my five pounds back if the badge came up for auction in an Antiques Road Trip. I never heard anything from the FSLP until recently, when they found my name and address in a file and wanted to inform me that they were reforming and that a convention was being held in Aylesbury. I was somewhat curious, and I decided to give the convention a visit.

The convention was held in a large marquee, on a farmer's field just outside of Aylesbury. The tent had been used the week before, for the farmer's daughter's wedding. I suspected that neither the local council nor the police were aware of this discreet convention. Security for entry into the tent was very tight. Membership cards had to be shown, tickets were paid for and then we had to sign in. It was very clearly pointed out that this was a private event.

As I entered the tent, I was surprised to see the mixture of people. Husbands and wives, girls with their boyfriends and a large number of single men. There were stalls around the marquee dealing with penis hygiene and others offering various creams and lubricants. There were magazines and DVDs for all tastes. At the end of the tent was a makeshift stage, with tables and chairs surrounding it.

I stood at the back surveying the scene when a rather camp man called Clive walked on to the stage. He was evidently the compere for the afternoon. He welcomed all to the convention and informed us that the competition was to begin. What competition? I thought. Silly! it was a penis convention. What sort of competition did I think it would be? Then to my horror, I had the ghastly thought that I'd have to participate. I was, therefore, much relieved when Clive produced a list and started calling participants on to the stage. Husbands left their wives; girlfriends kissed their boyfriends and wished them good luck. The single men were called up and strutted onto the stage with professional confidence.

All the men went behind a screen to prepare themselves while the judges came onto the stage. Three men. One with a tape measure, one with a clipboard to write the statistics and a third man to oversee that everything was correct and in order. When all was settled, Clive called out the name of the first contestant. John from Barnsley, with his proudly erect eight incher. The man with the tape measured John's impressive piece of manhood and the man with the clipboard wrote the details down.

What I was taken back by was the audiences' reaction. The men left in the audience smirked and made lewd comments, but the women screamed like teenagers at a pop concert. They screamed even louder when John was asked to perform his act, which was swinging his penis around in a circular motion, an action I think is called windmilling.

Malcom from Norwich was next. Again, hysterical screams. His party piece was to keep his pants on, pull out his pockets and declare it was the elephant with his cock acting as a trunk. My favourite act came towards the end of the show. Michael from Cheltenham. He treated us to a ventriloquist turn where he spoke to his proud erection, which replied in a high-pitched voice.

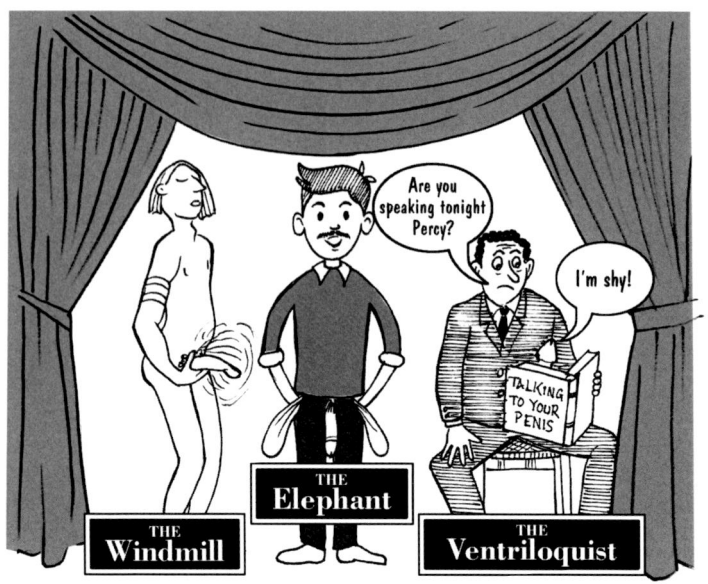

'Britain really has got talent!'

It was during this performance that I noticed at the side of the stage just near the steps leaning on to the rostrum, what appeared to be a boy in short trousers and a school uniform. No, I thought, that can't be right. I moved down to the front of the marquee to discover it wasn't a boy but a very small man about four-foot-high, dressed as a boy.

As the competition drew to a close, he jumped onto the stage and the whole audience laughed. He undid his fly and produced an extremely large penis, the type you can buy in a sex shop. The audience hooted with laughter, but I couldn't help reflecting on that period in the Middle Ages when kings and barons would have dwarves and deformed people perform for them. I had never subscribed to the PC movement, but even for me this was going too far. It no sooner started than it finished, with Clive asking for decorum as tea was served.

That was to me the highlight and the funniest part of the day. Three ladies from the local WI trundled in with a trolley and unloaded pots of tea, sandwiches and cakes on the trestle table, which previously had housed lubricants and sex toys. I suspect that the lovely ladies from the WI thought the afternoon was some form of talent competition or a country dancing convention. Everyone in the tent helped themselves to tea and a long chocolate eclair, and then stood around talking. I decided that I really didn't want to chat with the other people and was about to leave the marquee when Clive came up to me.

"I saw you standing by yourself," he said. "So, what did you make of it?"

I felt myself stuttering out a reply. "Not quite what I expected."

"What did you expect?" challenged Clive. I didn't know what to say, but I was saved by the bell. "Too late," said Clive, "duty calls."

And he made his way onto the stage to ask the three judges to return. When they were all assembled, he announced to the audience that presenting the prizes was none other than Leonardo DiCaprio. There was applause, a fanfare played from a CD player and in came Leonardo. Well let's be correct: a Leonardo look alike. In actual fact it was a boy from South Wales who looked uncannily like the movie star. What really took my breath away was that the women in the audience started screaming. They knew it wasn't Leonardo, but still they screamed. The whole thing was unreal and unpleasant to witness. It wasn't that the afternoon had been sexual or sexy. What it had been was debauched and decadent. It made one feel unclean.

I started to leave but I was stopped by the man on the door.

"Are you leaving?" he asked.
"Yes, I've a train to catch," I replied.

"Don't you want to know who won the competition?" he asked. "I've already made my own decision. The ventriloquist."

With that he laughed and handed me a leaflet for next year's convention in Harrogate.

I wonder what Agatha Christie would make of that.

On my journey home from Aylesbury, I thought of how the FSLP had in a way metamorphosed itself from a silly juvenile organisation, which I had joined over fifty years ago for a joke, into a sort of national 'swingers club'. I wondered what the gay men would do among the heterosexual swingers, but then I thought that they were all in for the same thing and at least they all knew the size if not the quality of the merchandise.

It should be noted that engagement with this organisation can only be made through an already active member of the FSLP. So, if you want to look it up on the internet you will be searching in vain.

MALE STRIPPERS

Male stripping has become very popular over the last few decades, partly due to the film *The Full Monty*, and partly because these strippers became a feature of all-women gatherings and hen parties. For these evenings, the men usually come dressed in uniform and perform for the ladies, slowly discarding their attire. The men performing must, as well as having a good body, be reasonably well-endowed. There is one thing that they have to keep in check and that is an erection. It is against British law to perform in public naked with a full erection. I think the strippers usually perform in such a way as to make the penis flaccid but not hard, and thus they excite the ladies.

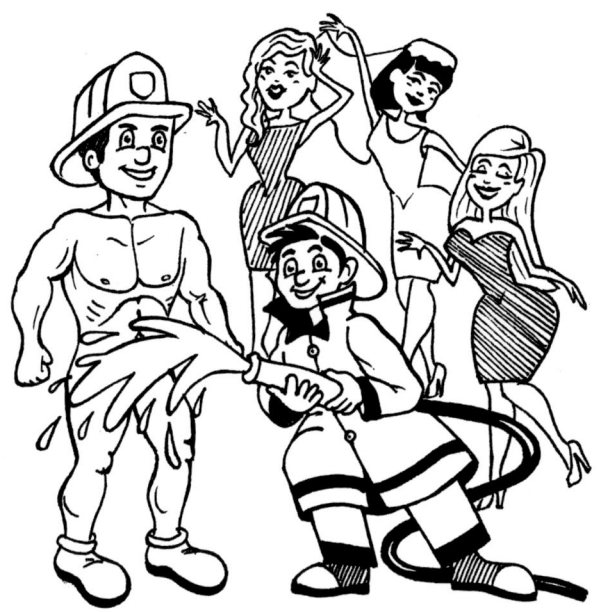

'Don't worry Sam, I've got your manhood covered'

RANDOM FACT

According to a study, on average, the penis of the homosexual man is larger than the average penis of the heterosexual man – 6.32 inches compared to 5.99 inches in length.

MEN'S NEED TO ENHANCE THEIR PENIS

In today's world it seems that men desire to enlarge their penis. I remember seeing the glass tube with a rubber pump sucking air out of the tube and stretching the inserted penis. I always thought that the result was never really worth the effort. A slightly longer, red, deformed penis – I cannot possibly see how that would be desirable. But now technology appears to have broken new grounds in the area of the developed penis culture. In 2019, the most-watched episode in Dragon's Den history showed brothers Mark and Dave Williams winning over the panel with their new wonder drug that would enhance and enlarge the male sexual organ. The claim was quite amazing.

Grow penis up to 2.6" in 1 month.
Grow penis up to 1" in the first week.
Improve the satisfaction of your partners.
Increase the length of time for an erection.
Increase sex drive and sexual confidence.

Clinical trials certainly appeared to support the boys' claim and they have some major personalities such as Mark McLean and Clint Eastwood promoting the product.
I have to say I remain sceptical.

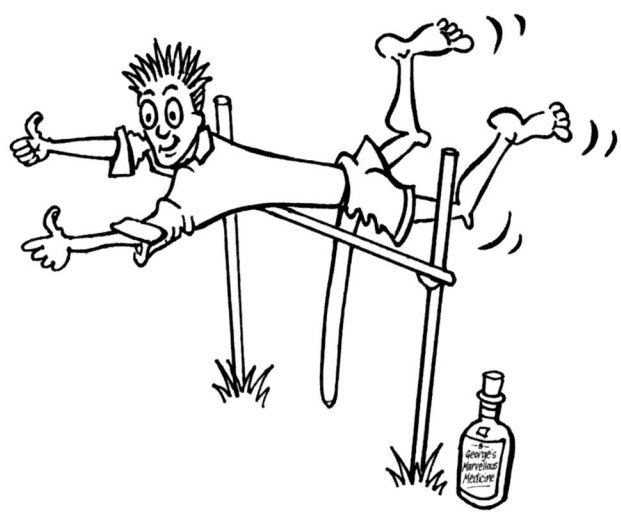

'I only thought this happened in Roald Dahl'

A SHORT SCENE

I wrote this short scene to be performed at our local Methodist thanksgiving service. Surprisingly, it was rejected.

MARY AND DAVE ARE IN BED

Mary: Dave, I had the girls from down the street in for tea this afternoon.
Dave: That must have been nice.
Mary: They started discussing their sex lives.
Dave: Was it interesting?
Mary: Well yes. They all said how exciting and stimulating it was, then they asked what my sex life was like, and I said it was not so much sex as virginal resuscitation. Deidre said that your penis couldn't be that big. *Big,* I said – *put it this way: Deidre,* I said *his cock needs its own zip code.*

They all laughed and then started to discuss the celebrations down the street for the Queen's Jubilee. They discussed the flags and bunting they were putting up.

When it got to me, so I said, "Dave will erect his flagpole and when he hoists his Jolly Roger, the whole street will know they're in for a good time."

Daft Liz then chipped in with, "Is Dave really that big?" I told her that when Dave has an erection, he has to have a blood transfusion to keep his blood circulating.

She then said that her husband only has a small one, and that she'd like to be with a man with a real battleship between his legs.

I said to her, "It's okay while the ship's at sea. The trouble comes when it wants to come into the harbour." I then showed them a photo of you last year on holiday in your bathing trunks and they all left in silence.

Tales of the Unexpected

Over many years I have been told some wonderful stories. The following stories are true if somewhat embellished for theatrical purposes. I called it Tales of the Unexpected but maybe it would be better called 'Cock Tales' or 'Short Stories of Long Dongs'.

Hey! Look What I've Got!

Young Brian Norris was only eleven years of age and was the proud possessor of a huge penis. It had started growing when he was eight and it was now well over six inches. Brian attended a junior school where all the other boys hadn't even reached puberty. Brian wasn't embarrassed with his over-sized cock, though he did wear a jock strap for games in case it dropped out from under his shorts, Brian was proud of what he had between his legs, and sitting at the back of the class he would often flash it, to see the look of shock-horror on the other kids' faces.

One day Mr. Perkins, his form master, walked into the room while young Brian had it out. It didn't register with Mr. Perkins what it was and he simply said, "Put that rubber thing away before I confiscate it."

Now, that would have been an interesting confiscation.

I Spy With My Little Eye

Bob Greenwood was gay; he was also the possessor of a huge monster. It was Bob's weekly ritual to go to the public convenience in the park every Saturday night at eleven-thirty p.m. with a flask of Heinz chicken soup, He would then lodge himself in a cubicle where he would stay till one-thirty a.m. drinking his soup and waiting for whoever came into the cubicle next to him. He used to say it was rather like fishing, waiting for the fish to swim by.

On the Saturday in question, what appeared to be a rather nice young man came into the cubicle next to Bob. After a while Bob pushed his man of war through the hole in the wall. The young man at the other side started giving it oral satisfaction and it grew, and it grew, and it grew. The young man, having satisfied himself on what must have been a tasty meal, left. Bob tried to withdraw himself, but the end of the penis had grown so big that he was unable to pull his weapon out.

Bob had to stay there while there was sufficient shrinkage. He said it felt like hours, I doubt if it was more than a minute. However, once released Bob was able to retrieve his friend and leave the toilet with his flask still full of Heinz chicken soup.

Oh! What A Big One!

Elspeth Brown was a great friend of mine. She was an editor for Harper's Bazaar. She was very smart, very sophisticated, and rather camp. She lived in South Kensington, not far from Harrods. She tells the story of how one day she was taking a short cut through a passageway that leads onto Kensington High Street, when this flasher jumped out at her with a huge cock.

"Hey Mrs give us a wank!"

Elspeth showed great presence of mind. She explained to the man that she was somewhat short-sighted and proceeded to put on her glasses. She then looked down at the man's proud erection.

She looked up and said, "I'm really sorry but I'm in a hurry, got a meeting to attend. But if you're here when I return I'll finish you off." She then continued her journey down the passage. The poor flasher was completely deflated.

The Wedding Present

Muriel Graham had been a spinster for fifty-eight years. She hated the term spinster and was thrilled when she agreed to marry Albert Wilkinson. Now poor Muriel had never seen a penis since she had seen her brothers at the age of five. Albert had failed to tell her of the monster that lurked within his pants. On the wedding night Muriel was naturally a little nervous, a virgin at fifty-eight, what was she to expect? Well she didn't expect to see what her eyes fell upon. Albert stood there proud as could be. Muriel grabbed the side of the bed, started to hyperventilate and then collapsed. She came round in St James's hospital in Leeds.

She was still traumatised by what she had seen, and she decided that she would have preferred to remain a spinster than to face that monster every night.

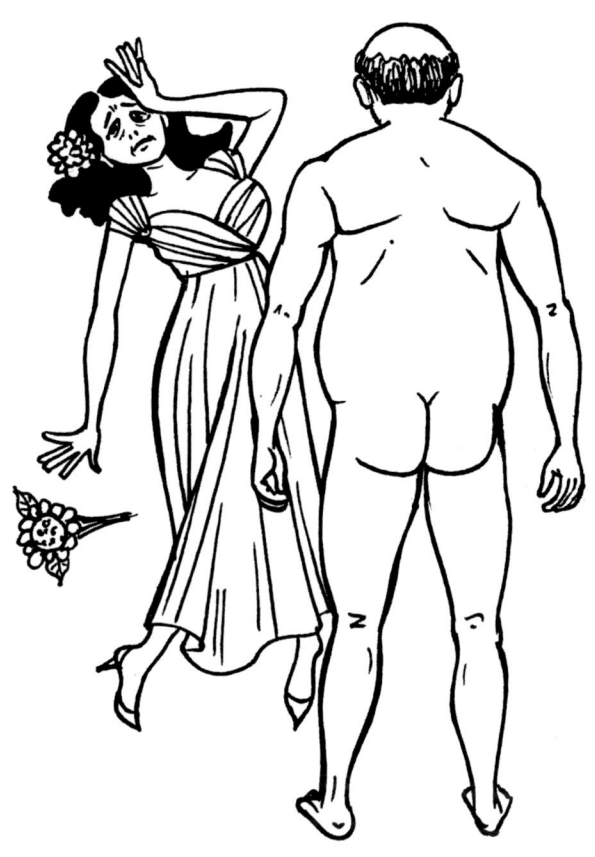

'I thought you'd be pleased'

PERFORMANCE ART

Leonard Whiting was definitely gay. He was what my mother would describe as a cissy. He was very feminine in both his manner, his voice, and his dress. Leonard was also small and very slight in build. He was, however, the possessor of an enormous penis, which caused him great distress.

He used to say, "Look at me; I'm a right fairy and yet I have a cock the size which would suit a builder or a lorry driver."

I used to say to him, "Never mind, Leonard, there's nothing you can do about it. Be proud of it, make it a feature of your body rather than hide it."

He seemed to understand what I said, but I feel he went slightly off-message, for I met him a few weeks later. I asked him how he'd got on. He told me he'd made it a feature of his personal property.

"How?" I asked, puzzled.

He then explained that with bright red lipstick he'd painted the end of his penis (that part in popular street culture that's called the policeman's helmet) and then had decorated the shaft with flowers.

"Well," I said, "it may not do anything for your sex life, but you may win this year's Turner Prize with it."

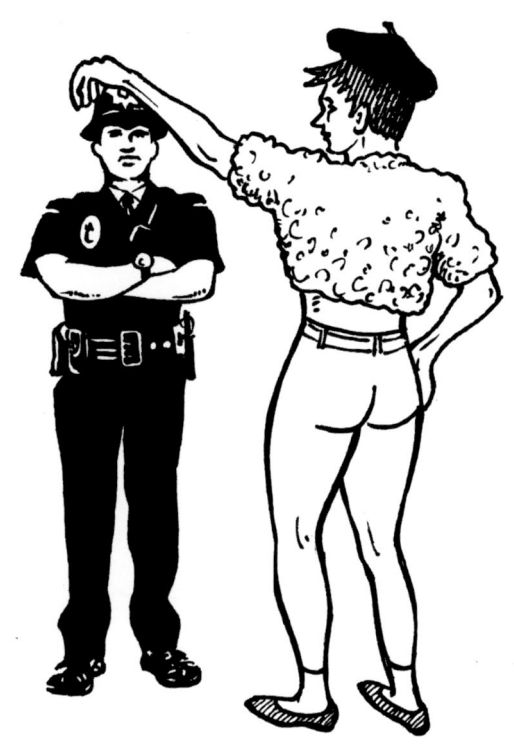

'But officer I am not a flasher, I am like Banksy expressing 'My work of art' to the world.'

MORE IS BETTER

Maisie who lived down Coltman Street and was a great friend of Edna Blunt loved cocks, of that there was no doubt. Whatever boy she went out with, she would ask him the size of his penis. It would have to be, she explained, at least 7 inches long before she would entertain it. She used to say, 'It's not just quality but quantity.' Some of the boys didn't know their size, so she would give them a tape measure and tell them to go into the bathroom and measure themselves.

I said to her, "Isn't that rather insensitive?"

"Yes," she replied, "I suppose it is. But I know what I want, and I won't settle for less."

If she'd have given me a tape I would have told her exactly where to put it, and she would have missed my Golden Globe award.

THE DRAMA CLASS

This is one of my favourite stories, for it shows charm and innocence. I was a teacher at a junior school. Every Tuesday morning, I had my class in the school hall – a drama lesson. On this particular morning I'd divided the class into groups of four and they had to try, with my help, to devise a short play. It all worked very well, and I suggested to the children that they could do the play the next week but to bring some props from home to support their play. They all agreed and left the hall discussing what they would bring.

On the following Tuesday the children entered the hall with their props: bowls, toy guns and toy handcuffs. We then sat back to see the various groups. It all went fine until a group of four little girls stood up and announced that they were doing a bank robbery.

"That's fine," I said, "let's see what you've done with it."

We saw the robbers get into their car, we saw them get out of the car and acknowledge a policeman who was passing by.

They then burst into the bank where the cashier was and said, "Put 'em up."

And then they produced a gun. But it wasn't a gun; it was a huge vibrator. I obviously allowed the group to finish, trying not to show my surprise. After the class was over, I asked where the little girl had got her 'gun'.

"Oh", she said, "it's my mam's. She keeps it in her drawer in the bedroom."

"Oh," I said, "well when you go home this evening, tell your mum I've seen it and that I will look forward to seeing her at parents' evening next week."

Needless to say, her mother never came to the parents' evening. What, however, struck me was the lack of reaction from the children? It was obvious that none of them had any idea what it was. Ah, the innocence of youth.

PUPPETRY OF THE PENIS

In 1970 I went to the Roundhouse in London to watch a show called *Oh! Calcutta!* where the cast of four boys and four girls performed an avant-garde revue completely naked. After the first five minutes, they dropped their towels. After the show, I felt, that it became rather prosaic and relied too heavily on sexual innuendo. That was in 1970. You think you've seen everything; how wrong you can be! Suddenly, something pops up to take you by surprise.

In 1997, a young Australian man, Simon Manley, decided to entertain his friends on New Year's Eve. He performed twelve tricks with his rather extended penis. It proved so popular that the following year he enrolled his friend, David Friend, to perform a comedy act, 'Dick Tricks', at the Melbourne International

Comedy Festival. This was a stand-up comedy act where they performed, to the amusement of the audience, genital origami. The act was so successful that under its new name, 'Puppetry of the Penis', it began a world tour of Europe, the USA and Great Britain, ending up with tumultuous applause and accolades at the Edinburgh Fringe Festival.

It was quite amazing what these two men could do with their genitalia. Something I would not recommend to the uninitiated. Simon Manley, who certainly lived up to his name, performed quite exotic sculptures with his length of artistic material.

The show was funny, amusing, but never really smutty or offensive. It was really a fait accompli. I think the world owes these two men a debt of gratitude for pulling down one of the last taboos in modern culture: male nudity. Up to 1998 we had seen much of the female in a state of undress, but by 2000 male nudity was becoming accepted on film. In 'Puppetry of the Penis' it was not just the exposure of a man's genitalia that was important; it was the fact that the two lads were so comfortable in their own bodies. It's a lesson we should all learn.

Psychological Notes on 'The Penis Being a Phallic Symbol'

Freud has always fascinated me, not because I believe in much of what he said, but because he came to such bizarre conclusions in a rather sexually repressed society.

A hundred years ago, Sigmund Freud published his papers entitled *The Interpretation of Dreams*. Freud's idea was that dreams were repressed sexual wishes that had to be repressed so as not to disturb the dreamer. All elongated objects, wrote Freud, such as sticks, tree trunks and umbrellas (the opening of these being compared to an erection) may stand for the male organ. The rubbing of a nail file on the nails is representative of masturbation, and boxes, cases, chests, cupboards and ovens represent the uterus. Stepladders or staircases, or walking up and down them, are representations of the sexual act. Quite wild stuff? and he a Victorian. The eminent psychologist Carl Jung completely dismissed Freud's theories as being far too simplistic.

"We dream," Jung maintained, "because dreaming is indispensable to our mental equilibrium. We create symbols because it is in our nature to do so. The penis," remarked Jung, "is itself a phallic symbol. It is also a symbol of life, death and rebirth."

Hence the widespread existence of phallic worship, claims Eugene Monick. It could be crudely sexual, such as the worship of Priapus, spiritual (the lingam of Shiva), regenerative (the maypole) or resurrective (the Djed Pillar of Osiris and the herma of ancient Greeks). I'm personally more attached to the naivety of Freud.

THE ROTENBERG CANNIBAL

I've always been a lover of crime fiction. Well this story isn't fiction, but boy is it scary.

Armin Meiwes had a desire to eat human flesh. He selected his victim on the internet and invited him to his home in Germany for a weekend (a weekend he would never return from). Discovering the victim had a rather large penis, he decided that this would be the best part to carve. He cut the penis off and he proceeded to fry it with shallots (rather a nice touch), and then served it and ate it while his victim was still alive. He then started cutting off other parts off his victim's body, which, to his surprise, killed the man. Armin was arrested for murder, which was then reduced to manslaughter, due to the fact that his victim was a willing participant. Armin served eight years in prison and then was released under licence. He now works in a Michelin-starred restaurant, where his famous dish, believe it or not, is *Cock au Vin*.

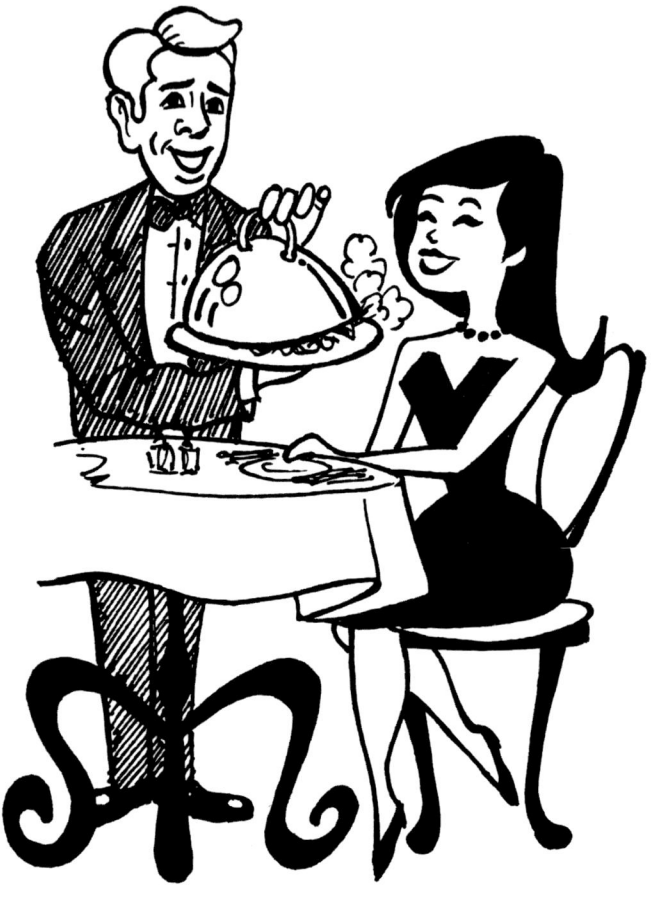

'This cock is covered in a cream and garlic sauce.
I am sure this Cock au Vin will be the best madam has ever tasted'.

I wasn't sure whether I should include this medical section in my book, but I decided to include it as readers could always omit it if they are bored.

AGS (Ageing Genitalia Syndrome)

To have sexual urges after the age of seventy is quite natural. However, the follow through of such urges can be severely restricted for the older man. In other words, the urge is willing, but the body isn't. After the age of seventy, men's physical prowess starts to take a nose-dive. The testicles drop to somewhere around the knees and erections become more problematic.

The problem is the pumping of the blood round the body, and the larger the penis the more stress there is on the pumping of the blood, leading to high blood pressure. Your doctor will no doubt put you on blood pressure tablets, which themselves will cause erectile problems. To continue taking poppers or Viagra, or both, can become very dangerous to your mortal being. In other words, there's a danger you may drop down dead while in the act of satisfying your limited needs. It's not to say that if you are over seventy that you are not able to get an erection, it's just that it won't be as hard and vibrant as it was in your twenties, and it won't be sustained for as long. (Read the paragraph on TA (testicular atrophy), age-related issues to testicular size).

Taking care of your penis

The penis can become sore with overuse. It can sustain red cuts and even bleed. Other books go into greater detail over this condition. My advice is simple: put some Savlon on the infected part and leave the bloody thing alone for a couple of days. A week's abstinence is not going to kill you.

A more serious problem, especially with large penises, is cumcrete. That is the solidifying of semen after it has been produced. Amounts of this are often left in the urethra and therefore it is recommended to drink a pint of water or lime juice directly after ejaculation (which is also good for your kidneys). This will flush out the penis and wash out any cumcrete that may still be lodged in the urethra. Not to remove the cumcrete can cause a build-up of semen, which in turn can cause a major problem in the future, as well as creating an unpleasant odour from the trapped urine that is unable to escape.

Cock and balls

I think it is essential to have large balls to accompany your large donger. There's nothing more absurd than to see a man swinging his large projectile and he only has small balls. The function of the testicle is to produce sperm. The average size of a man's testicle is about 4x3x2 centimetres and is oval-shaped. Most men have two testicles, also known as testes. It's common for one of a man's testicles to be a different size and for one to drop lower than the other. The small boy's testicles start to grow at the age of eight and complete their growth after the end of puberty.

Does the Size of the Testicle Affect Health?

In general, the size of the testicle does not directly affect health. However, some studies in animals suggests that testicle sizes may affect the amount of sperm the man produces.

In 2011 a study of sheep found that testicle size is directly related to the production of both testosterone and sperm. The study also suggested that a large testicle size may be more attractive to the females. However, researchers have yet to show whether these results apply to humans.

Hypogonadism

Some males have lower testosterone levels than others. Doctors usually refer to unusually low levels as testosterone deficiency or male *hypogonadism*. Typical symptoms can include:

- testicles that are smaller than average,
- less facial hair or less male-pattern body hair,
- growth of breast tissue,
- symptoms of *Klinefelter syndrome*, which is described below,
- *Hypogonadism* may develop during puberty.

Klinefelter Syndrome

Some males have small testicles as a result of *Klinefelter syndrome*. This results from being born with an extra X chromosome.

Klinefelter Syndrome can cause the following symptoms:
- undescended testicles,
- lower sperm activity,
- lower testosterone levels,
- certain female characteristics, and
- *infertility* in some cases.

As the body ages, the testicles grow smaller. The medical name for this is testicular atrophy (TA).

Age-related changes to testicular size

TA tends to be a gradual process. It may occur so slowly that the person doesn't notice the change in size. Other symptoms of TA can include reduced muscle mass and a gradual loss of sex drive. Old age is not something to look forward to.

Health concerns to look out for

Some health conditions can cause the testicles to shrink. If signs of this occurs, a person should seek medical treatment.

Examples that can cause the testicles to shrink include:
- sexually transmitted infections (STIs) such as syphilis and gonorrhoea,
- tuberculosis, mumps and some other viral infections, and
- trauma to the testicles.

Tips for Good Testicle Health

Males should examine their testicles at least once a month to check for any abnormalities. The check should take place after a hot bath or shower. You may want your partner to assist you in the examination. If so, make sure that their hands are warm, otherwise it will have the same effect as being plunged into the North Sea.

The American Urological Association provide the following tips for testicular examination:
- Perform the test standing up.
- Look for any swelling in the scrotum.
- Gently feel the scrotal sack to find one of the testicles.
- Gently roll the testicle between thumb and finger to feel its entire surface.
- Repeat the process with the other testicle.
- Check carefully for any lump or lumps.
- Swelling, soreness or pain.
- Change in size or texture.
- Change in firmness.

Testicular Cancer

Testicular cancer is a rare but highly treatable disease involving the testicles. If a doctor diagnoses and treats this cancer in its early stages, it is usually curable.

In Conclusion

So, if you have a big cock and big balls and the world is your oyster, though I'm not sure oysters are really an aphrodisiac even though they do contain large amounts of zinc and testosterone.

But why has the phallus become such an important symbol in our culture? Is it not the very fact that it is a symbol? As the cross is the symbol of faith, so the phallus is the symbol of life. Every male mammal in the animal kingdom has a penis. The larger the penis, the more hope the male has of attracting the female and thus ensuring the procreation of the species. Without this potent phallus there would be no life on earth, at least no life as we know it. It brings great joy and happiness to many families, though it can bring sadness and tragedy.

The human being, as we know, unlike all other animals, takes sex to a different level, a level of exotic pleasure. This can lead to stress, jealousy, and criminality. Once man has broken through what Freud describes as the psychological barrier of the psyche, he is prey to feelings that drive him on to unspeakable horrors; he becomes a predator: Peter Sutcliffe, Ian Brady, Fred West, Ian Huntley, and, in America, Jeffrey Dahmer were murderers and serial killers driven by the sexual power generated by the need to satisfy their fantasies. Though their thoughts are created in the brain, it is the phallus that drives this emotional need and climactic power.

In conclusion, I think it can be said that the large cock is not all it's cracked up to be. Certainly, women prefer a more average size. I think a 6-inch, well-formed penis is what should be aimed for. If you haven't got that, so what? Who the hell cares? Well you do obviously, otherwise you wouldn't have purchased this book.

GLOSSARY

- Journal of Urology.
- Freud's 'Interpretation of Dreams'.
- The American Urology Association.
- Medical News Today 24.9.2019.
- Psychological notes. 'Independent Newspaper'.
- 'The Penis itself as a phallic symbol'. Anthony Stevens 21.9.1998.
- 'Those About to Die'; Daniel P Mannix.

APPENDIX

Adolescence	17
Ageing genitalia syndrome	53
Albert, Prince	22, 23
Alexander the Great	12
American Urological Association	57
Anthony	12
Antiques Road Trip	34
Antisemitism	31, 32
Aphrodisiac	58
Apollo	10
Aristophanes	10
Aylesbury	33
Baker, Matt	22
Barnsley	35
Beckham, David	22
Bieber, Justin	33
Blind cock	53
Blood pressure	53
Bloom, Orlando	23
Brady, Ian	58
Brightman, Sarah	20
Bukkake	29
Charles, Prince	22
Chastity cage	9
Circumcised	32, 33
Cleopatra	12
Colosseum curtains	33
Commodus	11
Cottage	32

Craig, Daniel	22
Cumcrete	54
Czechoslovakia	32
Dahmer, Jeffrey	58
Daley, Tom	22
Deformed people	36
DiCaprio, Leonardo	37
Dick tricks	49
Djed pillar	51
Dragon's Den	40
Drury Lane drapes	11
Dwarf	36
Eastwood, Clint	40
Edinburgh Fringe Festival	50
Ejaculation	54
Elliot Minor	15, 16
Enhance the penis	41
Erectile problems	53
Esquivel Cabrera, Roberto	28
Falcon, Jonah Adam	28
Ferdinand VII.	24
Flynn, Errol	22
Formby, George	7, 15
Freud, Sigmund	50, 51
Friend, David	49
FSLP	33
Gay vernacular	10
Hasselhoff, David	23
Windmill	35
Hen party	38
Herma	51
Heterosexual	8
Holocaust	32
House of Casa dei Vetti	10
Huntley, Ian	58
Hypogonadism	55

Immaculate Conception	18
Interpretation of Dreams, the	50
Islamophobia	33
Isabel II of Spain	24
Jagger, Mick	22
Jewish	32
Journal of Urology	25, 59
Jung, Carl	51
Kafka, Franz	9
Klinefelter syndrome	55, 56
Lloyd Webber, Andrew	20, 22
Los Angeles	29
Male strippers	38
Manley, Simon	49
Marrow Song, The	14, 15
Maria Christina	24
Meiwes, Armin	51, 52
Melbourne International Comedy Festival	49
Micropenis	9
Middle Ages	13
Momoa, Jason	22
Monick, Eugene	51
Murphy, Eddie	23
Myths	25
Nazi Germany	32
Nero	11
Norton, James	22
Nureyev, Rudolph	22
Oh! Calcutta!	49
Osiris	51
Phallic worship	51
Phallus	61
Poland	32
Polari	32
Pompeii	11
Poppers	53

Pre-puberty	9
Priapus	10
Pritchard, A.J.	20, 21, 22
Puberty	15, 54
Puppetry of the penis	49
Ronaldo, Christiano	23
Round the Horn	32
Roundhouse	49
Russia	27, 32
Russel, Anna	30
Scott Fitzgerald	9
Sexual intercourse	17
Shiva	51
Spartacus	12
Sperm	54
Stryker, Jeff	29
Sutcliffe, Peter	58
Swingers' club	38
Testicle	55
Testicular atrophy	53
Testicular cancer	51
Testosterone	55
The Full Monty	38
Trump, Donald	19
Urethra	54
Vader the dolly	32
Ventriloquist	35, 36
Viagra	53
Victoria	24
West, Fred	55
West, Mae	24
Williams, Kenneth	32
With My Little Stick of Blackpool Rock	7, 15
World Data	8

The author

Hugh Nepis left school at sixteen to work in the display department of a large department store in Leeds. He worked there for four years until he was dismissed for arranging the stock in an inappropriate manner.

From there he went to London where he worked as an orderly at the Middlesex General Hospital. It was at this time he took up adult modelling and found he could earn more money with his clothes off than wearing a hospital uniform.

At Christmas 2019, he was given an American book on the problems of men who are cursed with a large penis. He felt that the book took the subject far too seriously so, when self-isolated during the Covid epidemic months, he decided to write his own account of life with a big donger. It turned out to be far more fun than endless days knitting or doing jigsaws.

novum ● PUBLISHER FOR NEW AUTHORS

The publisher

„ **He who stops getting better stops being good.**

This is the motto of novum publishing, and our focus is on finding new manuscripts, publishing them and offering long-term support to the authors.
Our publishing house was founded in 1997, and since then it has become THE expert for new authors and has won numerous awards.

Our editorial team will peruse each manuscript within a few weeks free of charge and without obligation.

You will find more information about
novum publishing and our books on the internet:

w w w . n o v u m - p u b l i s h i n g . c o . u k

Rate this book on our website!

www.novum-publishing.co.uk

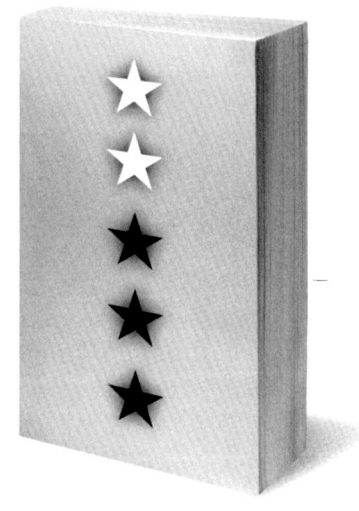